Ketogenic Diet Mistakes

You Wish You Knew

SARAH GIVENS

CONTENTS

Introduction

Are you having difficulty achieving or maintaining ketosis on your ketogenic diet? You're not alone! One of the main reasons many people give up on this type of eating plan is because they have trouble with the whole ketosis thing. That's a real shame because the benefits of a ketogenic diet are well known and growing with every new scientific study made public.

Eating to stay in ketosis is not complicated, but there are a lot of common mistakes and misconceptions that prevent people from reaping the full benefits.

If you've fallen victim to any of these errors, it's time to make a change. Don't turn away from ketogenic because 'it doesn't work'... because it does! Hundreds of thousands of people can attest to that.

The key is knowing how to get it working for you. The first step is making sure that you really understand what ketosis is all about and what things to expect. There's some complicated biochemistry involved with this. Many people need to go over the basics of ketosis several times before they truly understand the process.

The second step is avoiding some misunderstandings all too common with ketogenic diets. Making just one of the 'too much' or 'too little' mistakes can throw ketosis completely out of whack for you.

The final step is customizing the plan for your unique biochemistry, tweaking various things to find the best solution for you.

To discover the most common mistakes that people make when implementing a ketogenic diet and how to correct them, read on!

KETOSIS: THE PATH OF LEAST RESISTANCE

Although there are a number of variations on the ketogenic diet theme that are popular right now, it's nothing new, strange or unnatural. It's also not a 'fad' diet but rather a lifestyle change, a fundamental shift in your understanding of and relationship with food. The Ketogenic diet flies in the face of conventional 'wisdom' that we have been bombarded with from the government, schools, many nutritionists, and, unfortunately, from the medical community as well. So, it's important to thoroughly understand at least the basics of the process in order to make it work well for you. First, let's look at a little background information.

Our wonderfully adaptable human bodies have several ways to get the energy they need to do all the many and varied things that they do. They can burn either glucose or ketone bodies to accomplish this, and at different times we all utilize both of these sources of energy. Our brain uses a tremendous amount of energy and if it's deprived of glucose for 24-72 hours, it needs an alternative energy source in order for us to survive.

So, there are several 'back up' systems available. The protein in our muscle tissue can be metabolized, which is not a good option since our muscles would start to disappear making other tasks difficult, or our liver can convert fat into ketone bodies to be used as energy.

As Dr. Peter Attia, M.D., president of the Nutritional Science Initiative, explains it in his popular blog at The Eating Academy Web site, "The reason a starving person can live for 40-60 days is precisely because we can turn fat into ketones. If we had to rely on glucose, we'd die in a few days. If we could only rely on protein, we'd live a few more days but become completely debilitated with muscle wasting." (Attia, P. Ketosis-advantaged or misunderstood state? (Part 1), The Eating Academy, blog, n.d.)

Living, growing, and indeed thriving from ketone-based energy is not at all unnatural. Did you know that as newborns we are all in a state of ketosis? When breastfed, human infants burn ketones for energy in the form of breast milk. It's only with the introduction of carbohydrate-based food into our diet that we become primarily glucose-burners. A ketogenic diet was used in the early 1900s as a very effective treatment for epileptic seizures in children, although no one has scientifically figured out why it was effective. This treatment was largely replaced by drug-therapy in the 1930s, so no studies have been undertaken, unfortunately, although there is a resurgence of interest in it right now.

The 1950s saw the beginning of a change in people's eating habits. Convenience foods, fast food, prepackaged prepared food...they all began to have their effect on our nation's notion of 'supper', bringing far more carbs into our daily diet than we'd ever consumed before. In 1972, Dr. Robert Atkins set the food industry on its ear with the publication of Dr. Atkins' Diet Revolution. Atkins promoted a ketogenic diet, high fat and low carb, for weight loss and long-term good health. It did indeed prove to be a revolution, one that is still being fought over today.

The government with its 'food pyramid', the food and

agri-business industries, and the medical profession have advocated a low fat, high 'healthy' carb diet since the 1980s. During that same time we've seen a dramatic rise in obesity, diabetes, heart disease, and other so-called 'lifestyle' health problems, particularly in children. Both scientists and consumers have begun to question the accepted 'healthy' diet, and they've begun looking at alternatives and looking for support. "Where's the proof?" they've asked. "Where's the scientific evidence?" Those questions have led to many taking another look at ketogenic diets.

You are apparently one of them, one of the questioners and seekers of real answers, because you want to learn how to become an efficient ketone-burner. You want to set aside 'conventional wisdom' and try an alternative eating plan, but you've found that ketosis is somehow eluding you and you're not sure why.

When you take those steps to change from a glucose-burner to a ketone-burner, there are many small errors that can waylay your best efforts. You're dealing with intricate, complex biochemical reactions and processes, and it doesn't take much to misunderstand or mistakenly implement part of the plan. In this book, I'll examine those most common mistakes one by one, and I'll explain the difficulty and offer you some solutions.

So, let's get to it...ketosis and fat loss await you.

MISTAKE # 1: CALORIE MISCONCEPTIONS

A very common mistake in putting a ketogenic diet into practice is completely ignoring calories. That's not necessarily your error since many of the diet guidelines say 'don't worry about counting calories'. The good ones, however, should follow that with some additional information. Unfortunately, many people don't read that far, or they're basing their implementation of the eating protocol on information from a Twitter post or what their best friend told them. Do your homework and thoroughly understand the guidelines of the protocol that you've chosen to follow.

Ketogenic diets reverse the conventional—and highly publicized—'healthy diet'. The food pyramid tells us to eat high-carb, moderate lean meat, and low fat. Those carbs will be converted to glucose, which is our body's easiest way to get energy. Flip the formula around for ketosis to happen: high fat, moderate fatty protein, and low carbohydrates. Lacking the carbohydrates to make enough glucose, our bodies will convert the fats to ketone bodies, which will be burned for energy. Excess ketones will be sloughed off in urine.

It's true that the focus of any ketogenic diet is on macronutrients, not calories, and a high-fat diet in particular can be confusing to anyone who's tried to lose weight before.

Macronutrients (protein, carbohydrates, and fat) are discussed in terms of grams and percentages, not servings or calories, and it's easy to get confused about how much of something you should actually be eating. Grams and calories are not the same thing. You need to understand what your daily allotment of each macro really amounts to. On a ketogenic diet you will get a much higher percentage of your calories from fat and a much lower percentage from carbohydrates. That's how you enter ketosis and stay there: by giving your body fat to burn instead of the glucose that it would get from carbohydrates.

This doesn't mean, however, that you can consume unlimited calories and expect to lose pounds. Sorry, neither science nor basic math supports that. Your body has two basic and simple choices for dealing with the calories you consume: burn them or store them. If you eat more than you burn, the excess calories will be stored as fat. If you eat less than you use for energy, your body will call on your fat stores to make up for the deficit. Since calories seem to have become a taboo word when talking about a low-carb diet, it's easy to forget that simple energy equation. It's really easy to become lost in grams of protein, the glycemic index, macros, percentages, and whether you should count total carbs or net carbs, and forget that ultimately, calories DO matter.

According to Dr. Steve Phinney, a co-author of The New Atkins For a New You and The Art & Science of Low Carbohydrate Living:

"Don't count calories, although we ask you to use common sense. In the past, some individuals made the mistake of thinking they could stuff themselves with protein and fat and still lose weight. If the pounds are falling off, forget about calories. But if the scale won't budge or it seems to be taking you forever to lose, you might want to do a reality check, caloriewise." (Westman, Phinney, & Volek. The New Atkins For a New You, Touchstone, 2010)

I watched someone do this exact thing, thinking she was following the Atkins diet faithfully. She had a half-pound hamburger with cheese, bacon, tomato slice, and mayo (no bun) for lunch, but she didn't touch the French fries. Good, right? Unfortunately, not! The quantities were way off, even though the percentages might have been okay. She consumed two or three meals worth of protein at that one lunch. Add in breakfast and dinner and...oh, my! This type of calorie overload is not going to take weight (or body fat) off of a sedentary, middle-aged woman. No wonder she finally thought that the diet had failed her. She hadn't done her homework.

So, read Dr. Phinney's statement again, carefully. All the ketosis in the world can't help you if you consume way too many calories. Your daily quantities of protein and fat should fall within certain guidelines, based upon your lean body mass. Do the math and figure out what your recommended quantities are. Excess protein calories become body fat just as excess carb calories do. Use common sense and do a reality check on your calorie intake.

MISTAKE # 2: SCALE WATCHING

Trying to measure the success or failure of the ketogenic diet on a scale is one of the biggest mistakes keto newbies can make. Why? Because losing weight and losing fat are not the same thing! Weight is not your best indicator of fat loss, health, or general physical fitness. Think about it this way: what's the difference between your 280 lb. neighbor/boss/friend and a 280 lb. NFL linebacker? They weigh the same, don't they?

Muscle weighs more than fat; it's just heavier and denser. As we lose body fat, our muscle percentage increases, especially when we exercise in conjunction with the diet. So basically, the scale can register the same weight even though you've actually continued to lose body fat but you've also added some muscle mass. It's normal, and actually a good sign. Muscles burn calories. Fat doesn't. It just sits there. The more muscle you have, the more fat-burning resources you'll ultimately have available to you.

This shift from fat to muscle can also be a cause for the dreaded 'plateau', the evil bane of a dieter's existence. Days go by and the scale doesn't go down or, heaven help you, it goes up! What did I do wrong? Maybe nothing, so don't panic. There are a lot of complicated processes going on in your body and weight-loss plateaus are totally normal.

Expect them and try to wait them out. Some people will wake up one morning to find they've suddenly dropped several pounds. For others, the loss resumes more gradually but they notice nice changes in their measurements or clothes during the plateau period. Worrying and blaming yourself doesn't make it go away any faster. Most of the time, your body will break the plateau on its own in its own sweet time.

If the plateau lasts a while, there are various techniques to help jolt your system back into action again. Everyone has his own favorite method, but be warned, they don't all work for everyone. You'll find all sorts of advice on the Internet about how to break through a plateau. The two most popular involve opposite forms of attack.

Taking a 'cheat day' or 'cheat meal' can sometimes budge a plateau. This has to be done with caution, however. A 'cheat' simply involves allowing yourself some favorite foods that are normally not part of the diet protocol, in this case carbs. Increasing your carbohydrate consumption (within reason, please) can shake things up enough to get you back on fat-loss track, as well as satisfy any cravings you might be experiencing. Many people experience an upward jump in weight because of a 'cheat', and it can be a jump of several pounds. It is usually followed by either a drop in weight or a resumption of steady weight loss.

The other popular option for dealing with a plateau goes in the opposite direction. Drastically reducing your food consumption for a day can sometimes set the fat-loss train back in motion. Whether it's fasting, intermittent fasting or a mono-fruit day (eating nothing but apples, for instance), this type of shock to the system can get things back on track for many people.

There is, however, another form of 'scale watching' that can get in your way. That's obsessing over grams and percentages, weighing and measuring everything within an inch of its life, and trying to be 'perfect'. The food scale and the diet analyzing tools can undo you just as much as the bathroom scale.

Micromanaging your macronutrients, portions, and daily quotas can be very counterproductive. As a seasoned 'keto' veteran said, "A REALLY common mistake I see people making is that when they are first starting out, they try to write out a sample diet down to the EXACT number of each macronutrient they are shooting for. When you're first starting, try to just get the hang of it. Don't fret the details so much." (drandall90. Why Your Keto Diet Fails, bodybuilding.com, forums.)

Forget the scales! They're only tools, and inexact ones at that. They can lead you to lose sight of your true goals. How do you feel? How do your clothes fit? Is your waist smaller? Are you looking and feeling better? Are your measurements decreasing? Are your clothes fitting more loosely?

Yes? Then you're losing fat! It doesn't matter what any scale or nutrient calculator says.

MISTAKE #3: MEASURING KETONES

When you enter the state of ketosis, your body switches from depending on carbohydrates for fuel to burning fats for energy. As it metabolizes fat, your body makes molecules called ketones or ketone bodies.

As more fat is metabolized, more ketones are generated. Your body can use the ketones for energy, but there's one type of ketone body (acetone) that can't be used and it is sloughed off, mostly through the urine, the skin, and the breath. This is what is used to measure whether you're in ketosis and at what level you're burning ketones.

Measuring the level of ketones that you're excreting in your urine is one way to know that you're maintaining ketosis. Most sources recommend using ketone urine testing strips, better known by the brand name Ketostix. However, relying solely on ketone urine testing strips for determining ketosis is a common mistake.

They give you an instant and easy-to-read ketone level, but their accuracy can be affected by many things. There are also reasonably priced finger-pricking gadgets to measure ketones in your blood, which are much more accurate than urine analysis when done properly. Excreted ketone levels should hopefully be maintained between 0.5-3 mmol/L, with readings around 1.5-2 mmol/L being considered optimal.

However, many people who are new to a ketogenic diet become concerned or even obsessed about their 'numbers'. As Vicki Ewell of Kickin' Carb Clutter wrote: "If you're just starting a low carb diet and you don't want to mess around with ketone sticks, you don't have to. What the sticks measure is the amount of ketones your body is dumping because it can't use them.

For some people, that can be especially helpful for motivation, but there are other ways to tell if you are in ketosis." (Ewell, V. How Do I Know If I'm in Ketosis?, Kickin' Carb Clutter, blog, 1/28/12.)

The problem with the readings you get from ketone measuring devices is that you have to know how to interpret them. Ketone levels can be affected by many different factors, and those will, in turn, affect your 'numbers'. Your level of excreted ketones will vary naturally throughout the day, and your consumption of water, salt, etc., will also cause them to rise or fall. That's why many low-carb diet experts recommend that you forget about taking ketone levels unless you're having some particular problem.

Learning the signs of ketosis is far more workable and less stressful for many people. Some of the most common are:

- sweet, fruity or metal taste in the mouth (keto-breath)
- loss of food cravings
- weak odor of nail polish remover (acetone) on skin or breath
- increased mental clarity
- euphoria or a general feeling of wellbeing
- reduced appetite
- stronger-smelling urine
- more energy
- increased thirst

Most of the negative signs are temporary and will diminish as your body adapts to being in ketosis. Drink plenty of water and try chewing gum for the keto-breath. There are a few more negative reactions that some people experience, but I'll discuss those later in detail.

The other mistake that people make with the whole ketone issue, even health care professionals, is confusing nutritional ketosis (NK) with the far more serious condition, diabetic ketoacidosis (DKA). This confusion has been widespread since the Atkins Diet Revolution of 1972 and it unfortunately hasn't cleared up or gone away in spite of the scientific facts. So, some new ketogenic dieters feel that they need to constantly monitor their ketone levels to avoid developing DKA. Relax, it can't happen.

Dr. Peter Attia, M.D., explains it very clearly: "DKA is a pathologic (i.e., harmful) state that results from the complete or near absence of insulin. This occurs in the setting of type 1 diabetes or very end-stage type 2 diabetes. A person with a normal pancreas, regardless of how long they fast (including the fellow I reference above who fasted for 382 days!) or how much they restrict carbohydrates, can not enter DKA because even a trace amount of insulin will keep B-OHB levels below about 7 or 8 mm, well below the threshold to develop the pathologic acid-base abnormalities associated with DKA.

Let me reiterate, it is physiologically impossible to induce DKA in anyone that does not have T1D or very, very, very late-stage T2D with pancreatic 'burnout'." (Attia, P. Ketosis-advantaged or misunderstood state? (Part 1), The Eating Academy, blog, n.d.)

So, stop worrying so much about ketone levels. Measure them if you want to, but be more alert for the other signs of ketosis. Some people transition to ketosis fairly quickly, in a matter of days; others are more metabolically resistant to change and it takes longer, up to a couple of weeks. Watch for the signs, follow the macronutrient guidelines, check that you're not making some mistake in implementing the diet protocol, and...wait.

MISTAKE #4: CALCULATING CARBOHYDRATES

A very common newbie mistake is simply eating too many carbs. Not on purpose, of course, but not understanding the two stages of carbohydrate consumption can keep you from ketosis.

Carbohydrate intake on a ketogenic diet is divided into two phases: achieving ketosis and maintaining ketosis. The amount of carbohydrates that should be consumed in the two phases is different. To start, you need to get your body transitioned from burning glucose to utilizing fats, so your carbohydrate consumption needs to be really low, under 40 grams a day. That way your system doesn't have the carbs to convert to glucose, and it will be forced to switch to another source, ketones metabolized from fats.

Atkins actually recommends around 20 grams per day for the first month, which he calls 'induction', and many other sources recommend the same, 15-25 grams. Once your system has made the switch, then carbohydrates can be gradually increased and you'll still maintain ketosis.

How much is under 40 grams of carbs per day? Not much. Starchy veggies like potatoes, sweet veggies like carrots and corn, and beans/legumes are off the table, along with grains and breads. Just so you know, one small bagel has 48 grams of carbohydrate. In contrast, a stalk of celery is 1 gram of carbs; ½ cup of fresh green pepper has 2.2 grams; and ½ cup of chopped tomato gives you 8.6 grams of carbohydrates. Much better, but still you can see how a large lunch salad could easily take a big bite out of your day's allotment, and we haven't added in any carbs from things like cheese yet.

Green leafy veggies like lettuce, spinach, and arugula are really going to be the bulk of your carbs in the beginning. You'll quickly learn what gives you the most filling options while suiting your taste buds, but you still need to watch your portions. Dairy is great, but it has carbs along with the fat and you need to count them in as well.

In many ways, carbohydrates need to be your major concern, and it's an area where many people make errors. Your feelings of being 'full' have traditionally come from carbs; now you need to get that satisfaction from fats. That means that you really have to make your carbs count nutritionally. You'll need to get the biggest 'bang for your buck' out of your limited grams of carbohydrates. Nutritionally dense is what you're looking for—low carb grams that are high in vitamins and minerals. You can find lists of these on various Web sites, including Atkins' original recommended list. Pick your favorites, do your homework on them, and then watch your portions. Half a cup is less than many people think!

Another thing that many people overlook is that fruit is a carbohydrate. Healthier than bread, yes, but it's carbs all the same. Your body doesn't differentiate between 'good carbs' and 'bad carbs' when it's converting them to glucose. That's why it's a macronutrient. A carb is a carb is a carb, metabolically. And you can forget the glycemic index for now, too. It doesn't matter how quickly you convert the carbs to glucose. Ketosis is about not having carbs to convert at all.

Because fruit contains actual sugar along with its base carbs, you'll find that fruit is not recommended, especially for reaching ketosis. Here's why. Oranges are a wonderfully healthy food, but a very small orange (2.5 inch diameter) has 45 calories and 11 grams of carbohydrates. Most oranges that you buy are close to double that size! That's a full day's allotment of carbs in just one orange! Your system will grab those sugar carbs and go back to using glucose if it can, so you need to avoid or severely limit your fruit intake in order to get into ketosis.

Since fruit is encouraged on many other diet plans, this is an area where many people starting a ketogenic diet goof up. Save that orange for your 'cheat' day, if you take one every two weeks or so.

To get into ketosis and start burning fats for fuel, you need to really watch your carbs. Bulky, nutrient-dense vegetables should be your go-to carbs until you are fully transitioned to a ketogenic eating protocol.

MISTAKE #5: PROTEIN: THE GOOD, BAD, AND UGLY

Protein is an important macronutrient and it should make up about 25% of your daily food intake on a ketogenic diet. It can increase your feeling of 'fullness' because it takes longer for your digestive system to process protein than the other two macros. Since digestion burns calories, this is a win-win for fat loss.

You need to eat enough protein to maintain your system; otherwise, your body will scavenge it from muscle tissue. The necessary amount works out to about 0.7-0.9 grams per pound of body weight (1.5-2.0 g per kilo). That's less than many people think. Remember that half-pound burger I mentioned earlier? It had almost 40 grams of protein in it, without counting the cheese (14 g) and bacon (6 g). Since many women only need about 100 grams of protein per day, that adds up to 60% of the woman's allotment gone just for lunch. Once you add in the eggs and sausage at breakfast and the meat/fish for dinner, she's well over her 25% protein recommendation. There's a huge difference metabolically between 'enough' and 'too much'!

However, over-consumption of protein is an unfortunately common mistake made by people implementing Atkins or any other ketogenic diet. Quite apart from the 'excess calorie' possibility, your body has a nasty little surprise for you if you consume too much protein. It's a process called gluconeogenesis. Take a close look at the parts of that word: 'gluco' (glucose) 'neo' (new) 'genesis' (beginning). Doesn't sound good for reaching ketosis, does it?

Remember I told you earlier that your body would store excess protein calories as easily as it would store excess carb calories? What perhaps you don't know is that it will convert part of the extra protein into glucose to do so! This is not some weird thing that only happens with ketogenic diets. It goes on all the time and in all living creatures, as near as science can tell. Animals, plants, fungi, bacteria all use gluconeogenesis to maintain a certain minimum level of glucose in their system.

The liver will take any excess protein, break it down, and convert some of it to glucose, which is the body's preferred source of energy. Glucose is easier to metabolize than ketone bodies and your body likes to do things the easy way, just like the rest of us. It will latch onto that glucose and convert it to energy, preventing you from entering ketosis and burning ketones.

This is why excess protein is totally counterproductive on a ketogenic eating plan. It's a veritable Catch-22. You've virtually cut out carbs to deprive your system of easy access to glucose. You want to force it to burn ketones instead. Then, you give it so much protein that it can make its own glucose to utilize. You've created a vicious cycle that can completely undo your efforts to burn fat, and, if you don't check on your protein consumption, you'll never know. If your body can burn glucose, it will. Your mission is to keep it from getting ahold of glucose, if you want to achieve ketosis and start burning body fat.

Kris Gunnars of Authority Nutrition sums it up like this: "Low-carb dieters who eat a lot of lean animal foods can end up eating too much of it. When you eat more protein than your body needs, some of the amino acids in the protein will be turned into glucose via a process called gluconeogenesis.

This can become a problem on very low-carb, ketogenic diets and prevent your body from going into full-blown ketosis." (Gunnars, K. 5 Most Common Low-Carb Mistakes (and How To Avoid Them), Authority Nutrition, blog, n. d.)

Monitor your protein, staying within both your recommended grams per day and the 25% of total diet guideline. Choose the fattier cuts of meat, such as the 80/20 ground beef instead of the 95/5, and fattier fish like salmon, which will raise your fat intake as well as your satisfaction level, and save you money too.

Too much protein is one of the most common ketogenic diet errors. Many people mismanage this macronutrient, thinking 'more is better'. If you're having trouble getting into or maintaining ketosis, look carefully at this part of your implementation of the diet protocol.

Don't sabotage yourself.

MISTAKE #6: FAT PHOBIA

Years of hearing about the 'healthfulness' of low-fat diets has taken its toll on all of us. Many people have developed a 'fear of fats'. Even if they know that the whole low-fat thing was based on faulty scientific studies, the bombardment of anti-fat messages has left its mark. How many of us automatically reach for the low-fat yogurt, the 2% milk? This is not good on a ketogenic diet, and you need to get over it.

The most common ketogenic diet mistake is not eating enough fats. Ketogenic is a high-fat diet. Period. Fats should make up 65-75% of your daily food intake. It's what your liver will convert to ketones, then go looking for more in your stored body fat. Ketosis is fat burning. You know this, but still, a major mistake blocking many people from getting ketosis working for them is their fear of consuming fats.

Fat is the major macronutrient portion of a ketogenic diet. It's what will keep your energy up and prevent you from feeling hungry. If you're having trouble with ketosis, check how much and which fats you're eating.

First and foremost, you should be getting a lot of your fats along with your proteins. High-fat cuts of meat are the best thing you can eat on a ketogenic protocol. If you like organ meats like liver and kidney, go for it. They're loaded with all sorts of good, healthy stuff AND healthy fat (just watch your protein portions). You can devour that crispy chicken skin, and munch that crispy edge of fat on your steak. Seriously, we've been brainwashed to avoid eating these things, but it's time to reclaim the dietary fat!

What fats should you focus on? The best are saturated, monounsaturated, and Omega-3 fats. Avoid vegetable oil [corn or canola] and artificial trans fats, but be generous when adding butter, coconut oil, olive oil, and lard. Coconut oil is especially good for cooking because it doesn't break down when it's taken to high heat.

If you're not familiar with coconut oil, I'll clue you in that it doesn't make everything taste like coconuts. Liberally drizzle your veggies and add real butter to your sauces and meats. Rediscover the richness and the satisfaction of eating full fat dairy—yogurt, sour cream, milk, and heavy cream.

If you like to cook, investigate the classic French cooking style made famous by Julia Child and others. Many of the recipes are very keto-friendly if you replace the high-carb veggies (like potatoes) with lower-carb options (like cauliflower). The recipes use lots of butter, cream, and fatty meats superbly, and the taste is, of course, sublime.

Another way that people are keeping their fat percentage up is something called bulletproof coffee. Bulletproof coffee is all over the Internet, however, and just recently I saw a character on a weekly prime time drama drinking it. It's a combination of coffee, butter, and coconut oil, blended smooth, and often has a light touch of chocolate, vanilla, or cinnamon added in. The addition of the fats is said to turn plain coffee into a latte-like breakfast beverage that will give you energy and mental clarity for hours. It will also supply those much-needed fats to keep you in ketosis.

Many object to it because it's a nutrient deficient solution rather than nutrient dense, while others swear that once you try bulletproof, you'll never go back. You will need a blender with a glass container, or an immersion blender to make bulletproof coffee. You can't just let the fats melt in the coffee and float around on top. Well, you could but would you really want to?

Whichever way you choose to get your fats, it's paramount that you get enough of them. After years of having 'low fat is healthy' drilled into our heads, this is an area of radical change for most people. It's also a very common mistake on ketogenic diets.

If you're having trouble with ketosis, you may just need to get over your fat phobia and up your fat intake.

MISTAKE #7: REAL FOOD VS. FAKE FOOD

Another common mistake on ketogenic diets is not eating real food. What is meant by real: not coming from a can or a box. Just because Velveeta™ cheese is high in fat does not mean you should be eating it. This may seem obvious, but there are a lot of products and recipes out there that will lead you astray. Real food is a necessity to achieve and maintain ketosis and fat loss for several reasons.

Ketogenic eating focuses on three macronutrients: protein, carbohydrates, and fat. There is another layer of nutrition: the micronutrients. Some of these are very important in your ketogenic diet, and they'll be dealt with on their own later. As a group, micronutrients are the smaller building blocks that your body needs to carry on its various tasks. Many of these are the vitamins and minerals that you're already familiar with. Processed foods are often lacking these due to processing, so food companies add them back in artificially. Then the food can be called 'enriched'.

The problem with this is that what's replaced is only the major nutrients, the ones we know a lot about like iron. There's a whole substrata of tiny nutrients, some still unidentified, that get lost or destroyed in this process. Many of them play a necessary role in helping our body to use the major nutrients we're giving it, even if science hasn't yet identified that role. We need them. It's that simple. Processing takes them away. It's why your daily multivitamin can't replace healthy eating habits. There's a lot more to a carrot than fiber, carbs, and Vitamin D!

Another reason you need to focus on real food is that there are a lot of traps for the unwary ketogenic dieter out there, and they'll undo your efforts to get into ketosis and lose fat. First, the food industry has begun tailoring product labels to appeal to the most popular current diet trends. The terms they use have no legal meaning, so they can toss them around at will. 'Low-carb' bread? You know there's no bread on a ketogenic diet, but that 'low-carb' might tempt you to think it's OK. I mean, just a few slices, right? It's a slippery slope.

Learn your ketogenic recommended foods, print a list, and take it with you to the store. Take a good look around the grocery store, especially the diet and health food sections, and you'll be amazed at the number of 'low-carb' things you'll find that are nowhere close to being on your keto list! Sticking with real food from the perimeter of the store will help keep you from being suckered in.

The Internet is rife with recipes for ketogenic diets at the moment, and many of these are both helpful and delicious. They can give you fresh ideas, introduce you to new ketogenic foods, and help you to keep your meals interesting. There is, however, a tricky underside. I just saw a recipe (with photo) for 'keto-friendly' quesadillas. Really? I love quesadillas, so I checked it out and, unfortunately, found it wasn't 'keto-friendly' at all. One soft taco/fajita-sized tortilla has 29 grams of carbohydrates—that's a keto-killer right there. Darn! It might be a wonderful quesadilla recipe, but it has no place on a ketogenic meal menu. You have to beware of recipes that have just slapped a key word on them to get more 'hits'. Again, learn your ketogenic foods and guidelines or your road to ketosis will be washed out.

I've hinted at the final reason you need to stick to real foods in the preceding paragraph. We all have foods that we love, and we're well aware that they're not part of our menu right now. We miss them and we may crave them when we start a ketogenic diet, but we should never try to 'fake' them. Part of successfully implementing a ketogenic diet and entering a state of ketosis is changing the way we view food. Controlling food for our own health and wellbeing is a fundamental change from being controlled by food. Mentally and emotionally, we need to separate from the old unhealthy foods as well as the old attitudes towards food, and real food helps us to do that much easier.

Does that mean I'll never have a quesadilla again? Not a chance. However, whenever I do decide to munch into it as a 'cheat', I'll know exactly what I'm doing and what the consequences may be for my state of ketosis...and it won't be until I know I'm in a steady maintenance state of ketosis.

MISTAKE #8: ELECTROLYTE BALANCING

Electrolytes are the calcium, magnesium, potassium, and sodium levels in your body. If they get out of balance, you won't feel or function well. When you begin a low carb diet, it's easy to let your electrolytes get out of whack, and this is a common ketogenic diet mistake.

Before your body turns to burning ketones directly for energy, it will use up a lot of the extra stored glycogen in your body. The problem with that is that each gram of glycogen takes 3-4 grams of water with it. So, in the first few days, you're going to lose a ton of water, which is one reason that your water intake of 3-4 quarts minimum daily is very important. When you lose water, it takes both sodium and potassium with it, flushing them out of your system, which causes an instant electrolyte imbalance.

Keeping your water intake high helps, but you need to replace the sodium and potassium as well. If you're getting your limited carbohydrates from fresh vegetables, that may be adequate to replace your potassium. The most common symptoms of low potassium are muscular. If you experience achiness or tiredness in your muscles or outright muscle cramps, especially at night, you may need to up your potassium. The other common reaction to low potassium is nausea. So, if you have those problems with no obvious cause for them, increase your potassium intake either through your diet or with a supplement.

Salt is the solution for low sodium, and we've been warned off of it by conventional diets, so many people have already decreased their normal daily consumption of salt. Salt is essential for maintaining your electrolyte balance, so use more salt! Symptoms of low sodium are similar to what you feel in excessive summer heat when you become dehydrated: headache, weakness, confusion, nausea, and muscle twitches or cramps. In fact, those involved in heavy physical labor in the summer heat often supplement their increased water intake with salt tablets to prevent electrolyte imbalance.

However, on a ketogenic diet, you shouldn't need quite that much sodium! Consciously adding more salt to your food may be sufficient, although many people add a cup or two of bouillon (beef, vegetable, or chicken) to their daily routine. Those little cubes give you an inexpensive hot broth with a nice supply of salt. They make a wonderful mid-morning or mid-afternoon energy boost with virtually no calories. Throw them into your cooking as well, and of course, stay away from reduced-sodium food products. You need more salt!

As mentioned earlier, you also need to be drinking at least 3-4 quarts of water daily in addition to your other beverages. This is often misunderstood by those new to low-carbohydrate eating. A very common misconception is that you need more water to flush out the extra ketones and avoid serious health issues (like DKA). You do need to consume a lot of water, it's true, but not for the reasons that many assume. Water is crucial to maintaining your electrolyte balance and, during the metabolic transition from glucose burning to ketone burning, you'll be losing more water than usual. It will need to be replaced.

Studies estimate that up to 75% of us are chronically

dehydrated to start with, so drinking enough water is doubly important. Did you know that the 'thirst' message is often misread by the brain as hunger? This leads many folks to snack when what their body really wants is water!

Due to this crucial need to keep your electrolytes in balance, especially when new to a ketogenic diet, you may want to cut back on caffeine as well. Your caffeine-laden soft drinks are already off the table because of their high carbohydrate (sugar) content. Put away your 'diet' sodas as well, since artificial sweeteners are known to interfere with achieving ketosis and can actually increase your sugar cravings. The caffeine in your tea and coffee can accelerate your water loss, so just keep an eye on that if you drink a lot of them, including iced tea.

The water loss from burning glycogen along with your increased water intake will have two consequences, particularly early in your ketogenic diet. First, you'll drop a chunk of weight early on --- mostly water, so don't expect things to continue at that rate --- and you will have a greatly increased number of bathroom trips.

Seriously, you'll be going a lot, so plan on it and expect it. Don't get alarmed. Think of it as peeing out fat, and although that's not what's really happening, it makes it a little easier to deal with. Your body will adapt in just a couple of days. Promise.

If ketosis is eluding you and you're experiencing any of the symptoms mentioned above, check that you're getting enough water, salt, and potassium. Maintaining a good electrolyte balance is key.

MISTAKE #9: NET CARBS VS. TOTAL CARBS

Although fiber is a carbohydrate, it is not digestible by humans. Unlike ruminants such as cows, we don't have the enzymes to properly digest it and derive any nutrients from it. This has led to the 'total carb vs. net carb' debate, which confuses many people who are trying to adopt a ketogenic diet. It's the reason you'll find some plans recommending <25 grams of carbs a day and others talking about 50-60 grams. It all depends on how you count your fiber.

If you look on a U. S. or Canadian food label, you'll find 'Total Carbohydrates' listed. Underneath that, it's broken down into 'Dietary Fiber' and 'Sugars'. Sometimes 'Dietary Fiber' has 'Soluble Fiber' subbed out from it, which only means that that amount of the fiber will dissolve in water. That's not important for the purposes of figuring out your carb intake, but counting (or not counting) the fiber is. If you subtract the fiber grams from the total carb grams, you get net carbs, which means the amount of carbs that your body can do something with.

To further confuse the issue, European and Australian food labels don't give you 'Total Carbs'. What they list as 'Carbohydrate' is net carbs, and they list the fiber separately. If you buy imported items, you need to check the label carefully so you know how to read the carb content!

You also need to know if your guidelines are referring to total carbs (which include the fiber) or net carbs, which don't. It doesn't really matter how you do this, but you need to be consistent with it and you need to know how you're supposed to count those carbs. If your plan suggests 50 grams of carbohydrate (meaning total carbohydrate) and you're counting net carbs...then you're getting way too many carbs! You will not get into ketosis that way because you're giving your body too many carbs (glucose).

The total carb/net carb confusion is an easy area to get lost in, and it throws many a ketogenic dieter off track. It's a very common mistake.

The other issue that comes up with fiber is its role in digestion. If you're eating green and leafy, you should get enough dietary fiber from the food you're eating. Sometimes, however, ketogenic dieters have some difficulty with constipation, particularly if they regularly ate a lot of fiber (think oatmeal, etc.) before starting a ketogenic diet.

There are several alternative solutions, and you may have to experiment to find the one that works for you. The first is to choose vegetable carbs that are naturally higher in fiber, such as cucumber and tomato. However, these are often higher in calories as well, so you can only increase them within limits. Since keto is a high-fat diet, quite a number of sources recommend increasing your fat intake. More water also helps a large number of people.

Others will add a fiber supplement to help prevent constipation problems. This is another area where you need to read labels carefully. A number of fiber supplements contain sugar, artificial sweeteners, or citric acid to make them more palatable. Those are all items to be avoided on a ketogenic diet.

Psyllium powder is good but not very tasty. BeneFiber is a product to look into because it's very fine in texture and has no taste, dissolving without notice into just about any food --- even your bulletproof morning coffee.

There are other sources that claim that the 'not enough fiber' cause for constipation is a modern myth dating from the early 1970s. A 2012 study led by K. S. Ho would appear to support that contention. "Our study shows a very strong correlation between improving constipation and its associated symptoms after stopping dietary fiber intake." (Ho, K. S. et al. 'Stopping or Reducing Dietary Fiber Intake Reduces Constipation and its Associated Symptoms', World Journal of Gastroenterology, Sept. 7, 2012)

A ketogenic diet can be high in nuts, crucifers (like broccoli and cauliflower), and full-fat dairy, all of which are difficult to digest and therefore may cause constipation. If you've added a lot of these to your diet, you may want to cut back on them and see how that works for you.

It just may be the increased percentage of fiber in your diet that's causing you difficulty.

MISTAKE #10: SPECIFIC FAT REQUIREMENTS

Your ketosis or fat-loss problems may be due to something your keto diet plan may not even have mentioned, MCTs. These tend either to be overlooked or to be explained in complex scientific detail beyond the reach of many new dieters. That's why not getting enough MCTs is a common ketogenic mistake.

MCT is short-speak for medium chain triglycerides, a form of fat. Fat molecules are composed of carbon atoms formed into chains. The most common fats, and the ones most familiar to you, are long chain triglycerides (LCTs), made up of 16 to 24 atoms. These are the ones that are digested, re-formed, and transported through your blood stream. They can end up stored as 'chub' if they're not used for energy.

"All fats, whether they be saturated or unsaturated, from a cow or from corn, contain the same number of calories. The medium-chain fatty acids (MCTs), however, are different. They contain a little less and actually yield fewer calories than other fats", says Bruce Fife, N. D., the author of The Healing Power of Coconut Oil. (Picadilly Books, 2000)

Medium chain triglycerides (MCTs) have only between 4

and 14 linked atoms and, most importantly, your body processes them differently than LCTs. They are not digested but instead go directly to the blood stream for transport to the liver. Once there, they are converted to ketone bodies and burned for energy through ketosis. They provide quick energy, and there's nowhere for your body to store them as 'fat supply' unless you over-consume calories, when some other processes would kick in.

In a 2008 study, two groups of overweight people were given the same diet over a period of 16 weeks. They ate the same food with only one difference, whether MCTs or olive oil provided their dietary fat. Surprisingly, the MCT group lost more weight and more fat than the group consuming 'healthy' olive oil. (St-Onge, MP, & A. Bosarge. 'Weight-loss diet that includes consumption of medium-chain triacylglycerol oil leads to a greater rate of weight and fat mass loss than does olive oil'. American Journal of Clinical Nutrition, March 2008.)

MCTs are found naturally in both coconut and palm oil, as well as in ghee, a type of clarified butter. They are also available as a supplement in either liquid or capsule form, and they've become very popular with endurance athletes as a quick energy source. MCTs have been shown to benefit patients with diabetes, heart disease, cancer, Alzheimer's, HIV, and cystic fibrosis. They can also be very helpful for those on a ketogenic diet, especially if weight/fat loss is your goal.

If you've wondered why keto recipes, even for bulletproof coffee, talk about coconut oil all the time, now you know. If you haven't switched to coconut oil yet, seriously consider it, or pick up some MCT oil as a supplement. Either way, make sure to get MCTs into your diet to help boost both your energy and your fat loss.

MISTAKE #11: ADAPTATION PERIOD

One very big, but unfortunately very common keto mistake, is not giving yourself enough time for your body to convert from glucose burner to ketone burner. Depending on the individual, this process can take anywhere from a couple of days to 3-4 weeks. Your body is primed and ready to burn glucose, with nice stores of all the right enzymes to do so. Suddenly, you're not giving it the raw materials to get glucose. It hasn't kept a large supply of ketone-burning enzymes on hand, and it has to try to get with the new system fast. You have to expect a few bumps along that road!

Dr. Michael R. Eades, M.D., explains it this way: "It would be like a Ford automobile factory changing in one day into a plant that made iPads. All the autoworkers would show up and be clueless as how to make an iPad. It would take a while—not to mention a lot of chaos—to get rid of the autoworkers and replace them with iPad workers.

In a way, that's kind of what's happening during the low-carb adaptation period. Over the first few days to few weeks of low-carb adaptation, your body is laying off the carbohydrate worker enzymes and building new fat worker enzymes. Once the workforce in your body is changed out, you start functioning properly on your new low-carb, higher-fat diet." (Eades, M. 'Tips & Tricks for Starting (or Re-

Starting) Low Carb Pt. 1', The Blog of Michael R. Eades, M. D., May 30, 2011)

The many possible physical symptoms associated with this switchover period have become known as 'low-carb flu'. Although a few lucky individuals never experience any of these negative symptoms, it's good to know what's happening and what to do about them if and when they do show up. Too many people panic, think low carb is killing them, and go back to their old, fat-producing eating habits. The low-carb flu is actually a good sign that your system is moving towards ketosis.

The name 'flu' was well chosen, because that's how you may feel: easily tired, achy, and a little fuzzy headed. Treat yourself gently, get as much sleep as you can, and keep your water and salt intake high. You may get terrible carb cravings that pounce on you out of nowhere; you need to ignore them. Eat some nuts or cheese and drink more water. The occasional headaches may have several causes. If you've been a caffeine or sugar junkie, you're probably in withdrawal. Both are highly addictive, and you need to grit your teeth and wait it out. It will go away.

Electrolyte imbalance can also be signaled by headaches, so check your water, salt, and potassium. When electrolytes get really imbalanced, people can even experience dizziness, panic, anxiety attacks, and even mild heart palpitations, particularly when they wake up in the morning. That's pretty rare, however, especially if you are implementing a keto diet properly and getting enough water and salt. Try getting what's called 'lite' salt, which is half sodium and half potassium. Magnesium also helps a lot with any anxiety symptoms.

For most people, the low-carb flu is relatively mild, easy to deal with, and lasts only a few days. You'll find that the symptoms may come and go throughout the day, as well as vary from day to day. Now you know what to expect, you can be prepared to deal with it.

While you're putting yourself through this physical adaptation, it's not a good idea to throw too many other changes at yourself. Don't begin an exercise routine until your body is back on track. Back off on your exercise routine if you already have one, just as you would with a real illness. Your body needs all the energy it can get to convert itself into a ketone furnace!

Most importantly, remember that you're now asking your body to get energy the 'hard' way, from ketones. It's not going to be thrilled about that in the beginning; it's gotten used to the 'easy' glucose-burning way.

So, when you kick its lazy butt into action, don't panic when it kicks back a little. Salt and water are your best defense against the 'low-carb flu'.

MISTAKE #12: FLEXIBILE DIETING

Following any diet rigidly and blindly is not a long-term proposition. You can cut calories, eat things you don't like, be hungry and miserable for only so long before you snap! Then comes a binge, the guilt, and the self-blame. This is why so many people ultimately fail at weight loss on any plan. They either give up, or they gain the weight back and then try a different plan. A lack of flexibility in eating not only heads you down the road to long-term fat-loss failure, but it also can stall your actual process of losing weight. Your metabolism will readjust to the new system of eating, and the fat-loss can   slow way down.

A lack of flexibility is a huge mistake that many well-meaning people make when following a ketogenic diet, especially for fat loss.   We all want the weight gone last week, and we'll sacrifice anything to achieve that. That's a very short-term point-of-view because it's not a lifestyle change. If you want to keep the weight off, you need to make a new way of eating part of your lifestyle, something you can comfortably continue forever. Flexibility is how you do that. There are several areas you need to be flexible in, so let's take them in order.

First, even in the initial transition stage of a ketogenic diet, there are a lot of food choices. You don't have to live off bulletproof coffee and lettuce! Find a good list of keto foods (there are many readily available) and then find things that you like. If they're on the higher end of the 'approved carb' list, that's OK. Work out the rest of your meals for the day around that. Make sure you include foods that you enjoy, and don't eat the same thing over and over. The next step in flexibility is to try some new foods. Maybe you'll love them, and maybe you'll hate them...and that's OK too! As I mentioned earlier, don't become obsessed with exact numbers when it comes to your allotment of macronutrients. These are guidelines, remember? A couple of grams off is not going to make or break anything. Get the hang of it, then you can tweak your numbers, especially if you're not maintaining ketosis.

The second area of flexibility is dealing with your mistakes. And, yes, you'll make them. You can fall down, stay pudgy, and give up, or you can face that goof-up and fight back. So, you were weak and ate a baked potato? There's no 'keto police', you know! Accept that the error might set you back a bit and climb back on the keto horse. You're human, and that's OK. As Dr. Barry Sears, a pioneer in biotechnology and author of The Zone has often said, "You are only as good as your last meal, and you will be only as good as your next meal." If you slip up at one meal, get back on track at the next one. A popular expression with keto dieters is 'keep calm and keto on'.

You will have cravings. You will have foods you really really miss, and you'll need to deal with that, not ignore it. Suppressing cravings for too long can lead you to binging. How you deal with them is a very personal decision. This is where the 'cheats' I talked about earlier come in. Some people can control themselves enough to do little cheats, say one bite of a brownie or three French fries. This satisfies them for several days until they do another little cheat. This works for some, particularly if they were never big carb/sugar eaters before starting keto.

Most people don't have that sort of self-control. Unfortunately, one bite of brownie and the whole pan ends up eaten. So, every 10-14 days they allow themselves a 'cheat' meal or even a 'cheat' day. As long as you don't really overeat calorie-wise, it won't set you back too much. Satisfying those cravings can make it much easier to continue within the diet guidelines afterwards. An added benefit is that it can help to reset your metabolism, and ultimately restart the fat-loss process. This works for many people, especially as a plateau-buster.

If you stay flexible with your food choices, your mistakes, and your cravings, you will eventually be able to maintain ketosis easily. Once you are keto-adapted, there are two nice side effects: your carb cravings decrease and your carb intake can increase a bit.

Until then, be flexible.

MISTAKE #13: SPECIFIC LIFESTYLE CHANGES

Another common mistake made by keto dieters that keeps them from experiencing success is that they don't make some of the lifestyle changes that need to go with any diet. The two biggest lifestyle errors involve stress and sleep.

Stress can hormonally block your fat-loss efforts, so it's important to take steps to manage it. Adapting to a ketogenic diet is stressful to your body during the transition period (see Adapting). Asking it to deal with outside stress at the same time is a little counterproductive. Being stressed puts your body into 'fight or flight' mode and hormones like cortisol are released. Cortisol worsens your metabolic rate by lowering your ability to burn fat. This is also very bad for your weight loss because a major side effect of elevated stress hormones is increased hunger and sugar/carb cravings. Maybe this is why so many offices have doughnuts in the break room?

To lower your stress levels (and stress hormones), consider yoga, meditation, or deep breathing. Take some time out every day to decompress. Take long walks, indulge a hobby, cuddle your pet/child, play sports, or just take some solitary 'you' time to help clear your mind.

The other lifestyle factor that affects weight loss is sleep, or rather a lack of sleep. Being even slightly sleep deprived can make you feel hungrier and less motivated to exercise. It also interferes with your ability to make good food choices. If you're not getting enough sleep, you will not get the results you want from your keto diet.

"Sleep deprivation has been shown to lower leptin (an appetite-suppressing hormone produced by fat cells, which is normally produced in abundance at night) and increase ghrelin (a hormone released by the stomach that stimulates hunger, which is also secreted at night but normally in lesser amounts)," says Vanessa Bennington, Nurse Practitioner. (Bennington, V. 'How Sleep Deprivation Fries Your Hormones, Your Immune System, and Your Brain', Breaking Muscle Web site, n.d.)

There are many tips to improve the quality of your sleep, and you've no doubt heard many of them. However, here's one that you may not be familiar with, which comes from a recent scientific study, and it affects many people. The 'blue light' emitted by electronic screens (TV, computer, game monitor, phone) stimulates something in your brain that interferes with sleep. The study is still working to try to determine the exact nature of the process, but the results were conclusive. People exposed to 'blue light' had more difficulty with getting good quality sleep. They recommend staying away from electronic screens for about an hour before bed.

Paying attention to both stress and sleep may be the keys you need to achieve ketosis and to unlock your fat-loss goals.

MISTAKE #14: EXERCISE REQUIREMENTS

You would think that the more the exercise, the better the fat-loss. Unfortunately, you would be wrong, and this is a common keto mistake. If you don't already have an established exercise routine, don't start one until after you have become keto-adapted. Now, I don't mean just sit around. Stick to taking a stroll or a leisurely bike ride around the neighborhood. Suddenly starting to jog 5 miles a day will only put a lot of additional stress on your body, and it might make any symptoms of the low-carb flu worse. Your body will steal energy from elsewhere to accommodate the jogging, putting even more stress on your system. Make one change at a time, and you'll find that once you're burning ketones you'll be able to start that exercise routine without a problem.

Many sources recommend that even long-established workouts be cut back or even stopped until keto-adaptation has taken place. Remember, one of the common normal reactions of the transition period is fatigue and tiring easily, which may make a strenuous workout a really bad idea. Overexertion can push your body into utilizing muscle for energy and throw your electrolytes out of balance, and that's not where you want to go. If you need to cut back on your workouts, don't worry that you'll 'lose ground'. Ketosis generally makes people feel more energetic, so you'll get right back into your routine once you've adapted. If you do continue with your workouts, expect decreased performance levels. This is normal while keto-adapting, although not everyone experiences it. Your performance will be back to normal in a few weeks and it should increase in the long run.

You may read about 'carbing up' on fitness sites, particularly bodybuilding ones. This is simply taking in extra carbs before a workout. Until you're in steady ketosis, don't even consider this. The extra carbs will actually function to keep you away from the state of ketosis! Once you've adapted, carbing up is something you'll need to do some homework on. It's good for some and not so good for others, depending on the particular form and level of exercise.

Low-intensity workouts, weight lifting, and interval training will all help to stimulate your metabolism, increase muscle mass, relieve stress, and release healthy hormones. It's important to remember that your goal with exercise is not really burning calories. The calories burned are generally insignificant and easily offset with a few extra bites of dinner. The value of workouts really lies in the other things they provide.

If you've begun a ketogenic diet and an exercise routine at the same time, back off a bit. Get into ketosis first and the exercise and muscle mass will come.

MISTAKE #15: EXPECTATIONS

The final, 'most common mistake' on a ketogenic diet is having unrealistic expectations. This is partially due to the large drop in weight that many people experience during the first week. When the scale shows you a loss of 5-15 pounds, that's great! But you need to remember that a lot of it is water. As your body burns the stores of glucose and glycogen, you're going to lose water weight. You'll also lose some bloating, giving you a leaner look almost immediately. That's one very motivating aspect of a ketogenic diet!

However, it's not realistic to expect things to continue at that rate. You can't figure that because you lost seven pounds the first week, you'll lose 28 in four weeks. Once you're body starts drawing on its fat stores, you will lose weight, but at a more normal, healthy rate. We've all read about the people with the super dramatic weight losses, but many of them were very overweight at the start. The closer you get to your 'healthy' weight and the more muscle you carry, the slower you'll lose actual weight. That's why those last few pounds (the final ten) can be real bugbears to shed!

You also have to do some math with the numbers you see bandied about. I know 'I lost 102 pounds in just a year' sounds very dramatic, but let's walk through the math. A year is 52 weeks, so 102 pounds divided by 52 weeks is 1.96.

That's just under 2 pounds/week. That's a reasonable expectation.

Weight loss also depends on calories so don't forget about them. You need an actual calorie deficit to lose weight. If you stay on 'maintenance' level calories, you'll lose fat with a ketogenic diet. To lose fat and weight, you need to keep a reasonable calorie deficit of 15-20% below your maintenance levels. Why did I throw that reasonable in there?

Because if you cut your caloric intake too far or too fast, your brain shrieks 'starvation' and frantically tries to prepare for the coming famine by storing fat! It throws your whole metabolism out of whack, and that's what happens with many people who are referred to as 'yo-yo dieters'.

When they finish a diet, their bodies try to prepare for the next famine by storing fat and the weight already lost just pops back on.

Slow and steady calorie reduction keeps your system from freaking out and becoming more of a 'fat storer'.

You also need to realize that your 'maintenance' levels will not remain static. As you lose weight and fat, the calories you need to stay at your current weight will decrease. Therefore, to continue losing weight, you will need to adjust your calories on an ongoing basis. Your macronutrient amounts will need readjustment as well. If you don't reevaluate the needs for your current weight, you'll end up consuming too much protein, carbs or calories, which will stall your weight loss and could cause you to actually start regaining weight. Don't blame ketosis! Monitor your levels!

The final word about expectations is something I've already mentioned. Since it's crucial to your long term success, it bears repeating.

'Expect to make mistakes.' Don't hold yourself to some

crazy high standard of perfection. You will goof up and you will slip off the wagon. Everyone does. Accept it and move on.

Success comes to those who are brave enough to climb right back on the keto wagon so they can resume their fat-loss journey.

FINAL THOUGHTS

We've discussed fifteen of the most common mistakes that people make when following a ketogenic diet protocol. If you're having difficulty reaching or maintaining ketosis or have been worried about 'low-carb flu' symptoms, see if you can identify an area where you might be making an error in implementation. Slight changes can reap huge benefits when you're dealing with something as complex as human biochemistry!

Following a ketogenic diet can bring you optimal fat loss as well as numerous improvements in your overall health, both short and long term. The evidence that this is indeed a 'healthier' way to eat than the traditional food pyramid continues to mount with each new scientific study published. Making keto a part of your lifestyle will enable you to reap the benefits of a healthier (and happier) 'you' for many years to come.

Most importantly, know your ketogenic plan. It doesn't matter whether you've chosen Atkins, paleo, primal or whatever, know what you're supposed to do. As you put the plan into practice, keep going back to reread the explanations behind the instructions. You'll understand things better every time you do, and that understanding will help you avoid many common mistakes so you can fully benefit from your ketogenic diet. Keep this book as a quick reference of the most common errors with keto and what to do about them.

With a little perseverance and a little knowledge , I know you will succeed on the ketogenic diet and see your dreams of fat loss and restored health finally realized.

ALL THE BEST,

Sara

ABOUT THE AUTHOR

Sara Givens is a nationally known nutrition and health expert. She is a best-selling author of several popular health and wellness books. She has over 13 years of experience working in clinics and gyms dealing with health, diet, and exercise.

She is best known for helping people get to the root causes of poor health, dysfunction, and weight loss by designing low-carbohydrate, low-sugar, grain-free diets for her clients.

Sara lives in Colorado with her husband, two children, and her beloved hound dog Malcolm.

29282239R00041